Menopause Renewal

Banish Symptoms and

Rediscover Your Youthful Vigor

Virgie W. Miller

COPYRIGHT

TABLE OF CONTENT

INTRODUCTION

Menopause signifies the start of a new chapter rather than the end of youth. It's a time of change, with menstrual cycles ending and a new chapter of personal development and self-discovery commencing. The goal of the book "Menopause Renewal" is to reframe menopause as an empowered and positive experience.

Defining Menopause: A Fresh Start

There are a lot of myths and mysteries surrounding menopause. Although it's widely believed to be a sign of aging, this book casts doubt on that idea. Menopause is portrayed in this context as a chance to start again and start over. It's about accepting the shifts, getting to know your body's new rhythms, and drawing power from the knowledge accumulated over many years of experience.

Empowerment through Knowledge and Action

"Menopause Renewal" seeks to give you authority. It offers a plethora of information on how to handle INTROthe menopause's physical and emotional shifts with poise and assurance. The book is an appeal to action, motivating readers to take charge of their health, nurture their well-being, and live their lives with a fresh zest and determination.

By the time you finish reading this book, you'll have a thorough grasp of menopause and the skills necessary to successfully manage its symptoms. You'll be prepared to face this inevitable change with hope and a strengthened sense of mastery over your health. This is where your path to regaining your young vitality begins—welcome to your menopause regeneration.

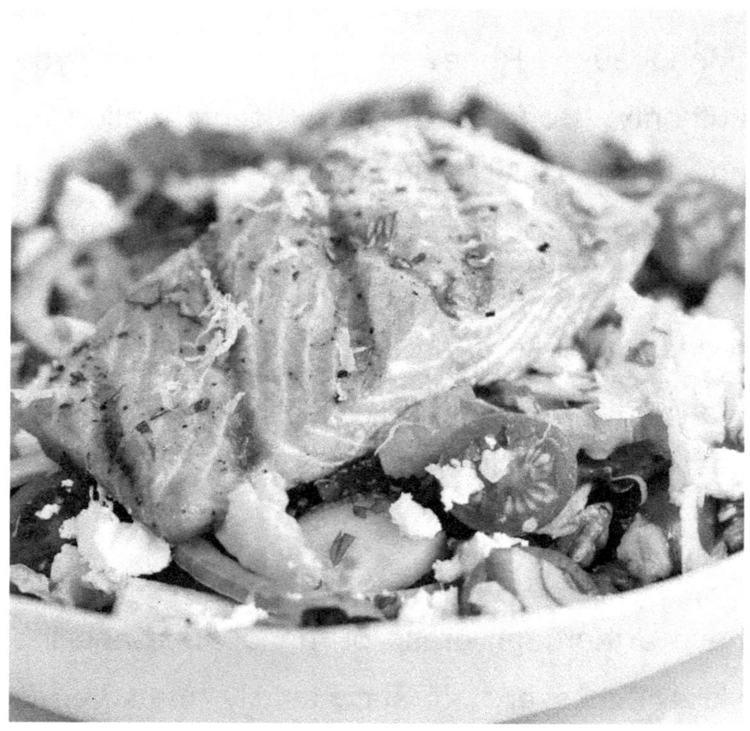

CHAPTER 1

THE SCIENCE OF CHANGE

Hormonal Changes: What's Going On Within

Women experience major hormonal changes in their bodies as menopause approaches. The hormones that control ovulation and menstruation, progesterone and estrogen, are gradually reduced by the ovaries. Hot flushes, nocturnal sweats, and mood swings are just a few of the symptoms that can result from this drop in hormone levels. It is essential to comprehend these changes to manage the transition successfully.

Estrogen: The Main Element

The hormone estrogen is essential to women's health. The heart, bones, and skin are just a few of the body parts that may be impacted by its reduction throughout menopause. Changes in these regions may result from lower estrogen levels, therefore it's critical to watch for and treat these consequences under medical supervision.

Progesterone: Leveling the Playbook

Another important hormone that functions in concert with estrogen is progesterone. Women may have irregular periods and trouble sleeping when their levels drop. Understanding the entire range of menopausal changes requires an understanding of the interaction between progesterone and estrogen.

Menopause Timeline: Perimenopause through Postmenopause

Perimenopause: The Start of the Transition

Hormonal variations become increasingly noticeable during the perimenopause, the time leading up to menopause. It may begin in her 40s or earlier and continue until menopause, which is the time when the ovaries cease producing eggs. Many women experience changes in the frequency and severity of their menstrual cycle during this phase.

The Official Milestone of Menopause

When there is no menstrual cycle for 12 consecutive months, the condition is formally diagnosed as menopause. This milestone might vary greatly from person to person, although it usually happens around the late 40s or early 50s. Even though it might cause symptoms that interfere with daily living, it is a normal biological process rather than a disease.

Postmenopause: An Emerging Health Stage

The phase after menopause is called postmenopause. For many women, the majority of menopausal symptoms subside when hormone levels settle at a new normal. On the other hand, postmenopausal women are more susceptible to certain medical disorders like osteoporosis and heart disease because of their decreased estrogen levels. To reduce these risks, it's critical to keep routine medical checkups and lead a healthy lifestyle.

A basic knowledge of the hormonal shifts that occur throughout menopause and the progression from perimenopause to postmenopause is given in this chapter. Women who possess this understanding can face menopause with awareness and be ready for the changes that lie ahead.

CHAPTER 2

INDICATIONS AND REMEDIES

Enumerating Symptoms, Common and Uncommon

Every woman's experience with menopause is different and can involve a range of symptoms, from minor to severe. Hot flashes, nocturnal sweats, mood swings, and insomnia are typical symptoms. Joint soreness, dry vagina, and changes in libido are examples of less common symptoms. To give a complete picture to the patient and the healthcare professional, it is critical to identify and record these events as they happen.

Making Sense of the Symptoms

The first step in treating symptoms is to comprehend them. Every symptom has a specific treatment plan, such as applying cooling sheets to alleviate night sweats or exercising frequently to improve mood and joint health.

Medical Methods for Managing Symptoms

Hormone replacement treatment (HRT), which raises estrogen levels to relieve many common symptoms, is a frequent medical intervention for menopause symptoms. HRT is not appropriate for everyone, therefore considerations about using it should be discussed with a healthcare provider.

Non-Hormonal Treatment Choices

Non-hormonal drugs can help manage some symptoms for persons who cannot take HRT or do not want to use it. For example, antidepressants can help with hot flashes and mood swings, while other drugs can help with cardiovascular health and bone loss.

Comprehensive Methods of Managing Symptoms

Many women find relief from medical conditions as well as via dietary adjustments and home cures. Menopausal symptoms can be lessened by regular exercise, a healthy diet, and stress-reduction strategies like meditation. Evening primrose oil and black cohosh are popular supplements for symptom relief, but their effectiveness varies, so consult a healthcare professional before using them.

Combining Techniques to Get the Best Relief

The most effective method for treating menopause symptoms is frequently a blend of conventional medicine and complementary therapies. Through close collaboration with healthcare providers and informed lifestyle decisions, women can determine the most efficient route to alleviate symptoms and enhance their general well-being throughout menopause.

CHAPTER 3

KNOWLEDGE OF NUTRITION

Hormone Balance Diet: Essential Nutrients and Foods

Diet is an important factor in maintaining hormonal balance throughout menopause. Including foods high in calcium, vitamin D, omega-3 fatty acids, phytoestrogens, and vitamin D can help maintain general health and control symptoms.

Plant-based substances called phytoestrogens function similarly to estrogen in the body. Good sources include foods like sesame seeds, flaxseeds, and soybeans. For healthy bones, dairy products, leafy greens, and fortified meals are excellent sources of calcium and vitamin D. Fish high in omega-3 fatty acids, such as mackerel and salmon, can help lower inflammation and elevate mood.

Diet Plan Specifically for Menopause

Nutrient-dense foods that support hormonal health and reduce symptoms are the main emphasis of a menopausal diet. Here are some recipes that use these ideas.

Day 1

Breakfast consists of a parfait of soy yogurt, berries, and walnuts.

Lunch is baked salmon and green salad with a vinaigrette of lemon and turmeric.

Meatballs made of beef and ground flaxseed for **dinner.**

Curry turmeric popcorn makes a **snack.**

Day 2

Berry and nutty flaxseed smoothie for **breakfast**.

Lunch: Mixed vegetable quinoa salad dressed with a lemon vinaigrette.

Dinner: Sweet potatoes and steamed broccoli paired with grilled chicken.

Snacks: Almond butter atop sliced apples.

Day 3

Overly hard-fried egg on top of whole wheat avocado toast for **breakfast**.

Lunch is a salad of spinach and kale topped with tomatoes, chickpeas, and balsamic dressing.

Dinner consists of baked cod over brown rice with roasted asparagus on the side.

Snacks: Greek yogurt topped with honey and chia seeds.

Recipe Books

Yogurt Parfait Made with Soy

Components

- 1 tub of soy yogurt
- half a cup of your favorite fruit
- 2-Tbsp chopped walnuts

Guidelines

- Arrange the soy yogurt in a layer at the base of a glass.
- Spread some berries on top.
- Add a little bit of walnut on top.

- Continue layering the ingredients until all of them are used.
- Present cold.

Salmon and Green Salad with Turmeric-Lemon Dressing

Ingredients

- 1/2 cup diced cucumber
- 1 medium tomato
- chopped spinach
- arugula
- romaine
- 1 tablespoon olive oil
- 1 tablespoon lemon juice
- 4 ounces of salmon fillet
- 2 tsp minced garlic
- To taste, add salt and pepper.

Guidelines

- Set the oven to 190°C, or 375°F.
- Transfer the salmon to a baking tray, sprinkle with salt and pepper, and bake for 15 to 20 minutes, or until it is cooked through.
- To make the dressing, combine the olive oil, lemon juice, garlic, and a tiny amount of salt and pepper in a small bowl.
- Combine the cucumber, tomato, and mixed greens with the dressing.
- Place the baked salmon on top of the salad and serve.

Soy and Flaxseed Smoothie

Ingredients

- 1 cup soy milk
- 1 tablespoon milled flaxseed
- One banana
- 1/2 cup of berry mixture

- One teaspoon of honey, if desired

Guidelines

- Fill a blender with all the ingredients.
- Process until smooth.
- Present right away.

Steamed Greens and Salmon

Ingredients

- 1 tablespoon olive oil
- 2 salmon filets
- 1 minced garlic clove
- Two cups of mixed greens (kale, Swiss chard, and spinach)
- To taste, add salt and pepper.

Guidelines

- Set the oven's temperature to 175°C/350°F.
- Transfer fish to a baking sheet, brush with olive oil, and sprinkle with salt, pepper, and garlic.
- Bake for twenty minutes, or until a fork can easily pierce the salmon.
- Steam greens for a soft texture.
- Present salmon with steaming greens as an accompaniment.

Rich in Calcium Yogurt Parfait

Components

- One cup of Greek yogurt
- 1/2 cup granola
- 1/2 cup sliced fresh strawberries
- 1 tablespoon chopped almonds

Guidelines

- Arrange a glass with half of the yogurt on top.
- Top with a layer of strawberries and then granola.
- Go through the layers again.
- Add chopped almonds on top.
- Savor as a snack or breakfast.

Chickpea and Spinach Curry:

Ingredients

- 1 tablespoon olive oil;
- 1 finely chopped onion
- 2 minced garlic cloves
- 1 teaspoon each of ground cumin and coriander
- Half a teaspoon of turmeric
- One can (14 ounces) of rinsed and drained chickpeas
- one can (14 ounces) of diced tomatoes

- Four cups of fresh spinach - Toppings of salt and pepper

Guidelines

- Heat the olive oil in a big pan over medium heat.
- Add the garlic and onion and sauté until tender.
- Cook for a further minute after adding the turmeric, coriander, and cumin.
- Include the tomatoes and chickpeas and boil.
- Add the spinach and heat until wilted after cooking for ten minutes.
- Add pepper and salt for seasoning.
- Accompany with naan bread or brown rice.

Quinoa Salad with Vegetable Combinations

Ingredients

- 2 cups water and 1 cup quinoa
- 1/4 cup chopped fresh parsley
- 1/4 cup lemon juice
- 1 diced red bell pepper
- 1 diced cucumber
- 1/2 red onion, finely chopped
- Two tsp olive oil
- To taste, add salt and pepper.

Guidelines

- Make sure to rinse the quinoa with cool water.
- Place the quinoa and water in a pot and bring to a boil.
- Simmer for fifteen minutes with a covered lid on low heat.

- Turn off the heat and allow it to stand for five minutes before fluffing with a fork.
- Combine the cooked quinoa, cucumber, red onion, red bell pepper, and parsley in a big bowl.
- To make the dressing, combine the lemon juice, olive oil, salt, and pepper in a small bowl.
- Drizzle the salad with the dressing and toss to mix.
- Before serving, let the food cool in the refrigerator for at least half an hour.

Berry and Walnut Oatmeal

Ingredients

- 1 cup rolled oats
- 2 cups water or milk
- 1/2 cup of mixed berries, either frozen or fresh
- 1/4 cup chopped walnuts

- 1 tablespoon maple syrup or honey
- An optional pinch of cinnamon

Guidelines

- In a saucepan, bring the milk or water to a boil.
- Add the oats and cook over low heat.
- Cook, stirring periodically, for five minutes.
- Take the oats off the stove as soon as they are tender and the liquid has been mostly absorbed.
- Add the cinnamon, honey or maple syrup, walnuts, and berries.
- For a filling and healthful start to the day, serve warm.

spinach and feta cheese omelette

Ingredients

- eggs
- spinach
- feta cheese
- olive oil
- salt
- pepper.

Guidelines

- In olive oil, sauté spinach; whisk in eggs; add spinach and crumbled feta; simmer until set; serve hot.

Stir-fried Tofu

Ingredients

- Sesame oil
- soy sauce
- ginger
- garlic
- bell peppers together with a mixture of veggies (carrots, broccoli, and bell peppers).

Directions

- Heat the tofu until it becomes golden, then add the veggies, ginger, and garlic.
- Stir in the soy sauce and sesame oil and cook until the veggies are soft. Serve over brown rice.

Salmon Salad

Ingredients

- Cucumber
- cherry tomatoes
- avocado
- mixed greens
- lemon vinaigrette.

Guidelines

- Serve cooked grilled salmon flake over mixed greens, garnish with sliced avocado, cherry tomatoes, and cucumber, and dress with lemon vinaigrette.

Quinoa Stir-Fry with Veggies

Ingredients

- Quinoa
- mixed veggies (carrots, snap peas, and bell peppers)
- tofu or chicken
- sesame oil, garlic
- soy sauce

Guidelines

- Prepare the quinoa as directed on the box
- add the cooked quinoa and soy sauce to a stir-fried mixture of mixed veggies and your preferred protein in garlic and sesame oil, and serve hot.

Watermelon Cucumber Salad

Ingredients

- Watermelon
- cucumber
- feta cheese
- lime juice
- mint leaves.

Guidelines

- Cut the cucumber and watermelon into cubes, add the crumbled feta cheese and broken mint leaves, squeeze in some lime juice, and serve cold.

Greek yogurt parfait

Ingredients

- Greek yogurt
- mixed berries (strawberries, blueberries, raspberries)
- granola

- honey

Guidelines

- In a glass, arrange Greek yogurt, granola, and mixed berries; top with honey and serve cold.

Lentil salad

Ingredients

- Cooked lentils
- chopped cucumbers
- cherry tomatoes, red onion
- feta cheese
- fresh parsley
- a lemon-tahini vinaigrette

Guidelines

- Place the lentils, cucumbers, tomatoes, red onion, and feta cheese in a bowl

- add the lemon-tahini dressing; mix well and serve. Garnish with fresh parsley.

Roasted Vegetables with Grilled Chicken

Ingredients

- Skinless
- boneless chicken breasts
- mixed veggies (onions, bell peppers, and zucchini); balsamic vinegar; garlic; and rosemary.

Guidelines

- Chicken should be marinated in olive oil, balsamic vinegar, garlic, and rosemary before being cooked on the grill.
- Serve roasted mixed vegetables with grilled chicken after tossing them with olive oil, garlic, salt, and pepper until they become soft.

Apple with Almond Butter

Ingredients:

- 1 apple (any variety you prefer)
- Almond butter
- Optional toppings: cinnamon, honey, granola, sliced almonds

Guiidelines

- Cut an apple into slices and top with a dollop of almond butter for a filling and healthful snack that's high in vitamins, fiber, and healthy fats.

Hummus with Veggie Sticks

Ingredients

- 2 chopped garlic cloves - 1 can (15 ounces) of drained and rinsed chickpeas - 2-3 tablespoons of tahini (sesame seed paste)
- Two tsp freshly squeezed lemon juice
- Two to three tsp extra virgin olive oil
- One teaspoon of ground flaxseeds, which are high in omega-3 fatty acids and may aid with menopausal symptoms
- Half a teaspoon of ground turmeric, which has anti-inflammatory qualities

- To taste salt - A variety of vegetables (carrots, cucumbers, bell peppers, celery, cherry tomatoes, etc.) for dipping

Guidelines:

- Place the chickpeas, tahini, minced garlic, lemon juice, ground flaxseeds, ground turmeric, and a small amount of salt in a food processor.
- Process the mixture until it's smooth, stopping occasionally to scrape down the bowl's edges.
- While the food processor is operating, add the olive oil little by little until the hummus has the consistency you want.

- After tasting the hummus, adjust the seasoning by adding extra salt or lemon juice, if preferred.
- Spoon the hummus onto a serving bowl and, if preferred, dress it with a little more olive oil.
- Wash and chop your assortment of vegetables into bite-sized pieces or sticks for dipping.
- Place the vegetable sticks around the hummus bowl and proceed to serve.
- Savor your satisfying and tasty snack—ideal for helping women through the menopause transition!

A blend of Herbal Tea

Components

- Chamomile
- Lavender Tea

Instructions

- Brew a calming tea infusion of chamomile and lavender to sip throughout the day for relaxation and hydration.

To support general well-being during menopause, keep an active lifestyle, pay attention to your body's signals of hunger and fullness, and emphasize self-care.

Recall that for individualized guidance catered to specific requirements and medical situations, speak with a licensed dietitian or other healthcare expert.

Simple, wholesome, and specifically crafted to maintain hormonal balance throughout menopause, these meals are meant to be enjoyed by all. Including them in your diet can help you transition more smoothly and maintain greater health.

CHAPTER 4

MENOPAUSE AND MOVEMENT

Exercise Plans for Increasing Bone Density, Strength, and Flexibility

The changes brought about by menopause may have an impact on a woman's bone density, flexibility, and strength. Developing a focused workout regimen can assist in reducing these impacts and enhancing general well-being.

Increasing Power

During the menopause, strength exercise is crucial. It aids in preserving muscular mass, which ages naturally. Exercises with body weight, free weights, or resistance bands work well. Exercises that strengthen the big muscular groups in the thighs and buttocks, including squats and lunges, are good for maintaining bone health.

Improving Adaptability

Stretching and yoga are two examples of flexibility activities that can increase joint range of motion and reduce the chance of injury. Stretching every day for all of the main muscle groups increases flexibility and has the potential to reduce stress.

Increasing Density of Bones

For strong bones, weight-bearing activities like jogging, walking, and stair climbing are essential. Engaging in these activities can promote bone growth and mitigate bone loss associated with menopause.

Customizing Your Workout Program: Examples

Every woman's experience with menopause is different, and her fitness routine should reflect this. These case studies show how fitness plans may be customized to meet the demands of each individual.

Case Study 1: The Journey of Jane

52-year-old Jane, who has a sedentary lifestyle, began to feel the signs of menopause and was worried about osteoporosis. Her exercise routine started off with low-impact exercises like brisk walking and progressively expanded to include twice-weekly strength training. Jane experienced more control over her menopausal symptoms as her bone density increased over time.

Case Study No. 2: Maria's Approach

Maria, a 49-year-old tennis enthusiast, observed a decline in her flexibility. She added yoga to her regimen and started practicing three times a week to address this. This enhanced both her flexibility and her game, demonstrating how individual motivations can influence fitness decisions.

These case studies show how highly customized fitness programs can improve quality of life and health outcomes during menopause. Women can design an exercise program that matches their lifestyle and takes care of their particular issues by learning the science underlying the changes and consulting with healthcare providers.

CHAPTER 5

MANAGING MENOPAUSE MINDSET

Supportive Therapies and Mental Health Issues

For many women, the menopause transition can be a mentally taxing time. Mood fluctuations, anxiety, and despair can result from fluctuating hormone levels. During this time, women frequently experience twice as many cases of depression. Supportive therapies are essential for the management of various mental health issues.

Complementary Therapies for Mental Health

During menopause, a variety of therapies can provide comfort and assistance. It is advised to employ cognitive behavioral therapy (CBT) to treat anxiety and depression, which are frequently linked to menopause. It is beneficial because it modifies harmful mental patterns and actions. Additional supportive therapies that help enhance mental health after menopause include group therapy, health coaching, and even marital assistance.

Cognitive techniques, meditation, and mindfulness

Accepting Meditation and Mindfulness

Two effective strategies for overcoming the psychological difficulties of menopause are mindfulness and meditation. Women who engage in these activities report feeling more present and less stressed, which helps lessen hot flashes and enhance their general quality of life. The 4-7-8 approach, boxed breathing, and deep breathing are a few easy yet powerful strategies to incorporate relaxation into daily life.

Cognitive Methods for Managing Symptoms

The goal of cognitive approaches is to enhance mental functions such as memory and concentration, which can be impacted by menopause. These include doing memory exercises, taking part in mentally stimulating activities, and treating cognitive issues with cognitive behavioral therapy (CBT). Women can better tolerate the mental fog that occasionally accompanies menopause by increasing their cognitive function.

This chapter describes the mental health issues that can come up during menopause as well as the different methods and treatments that can help women get through this change. Women can preserve emotional stability and mental clarity at this important stage of life by learning and applying these techniques.

CHAPTER 6

THE PATH OF EMOTIONS

Handling Emotional Upheaval and Mood Swings

A man going through menopause may endure mood swings and emotional upheaval, which can be an emotional rollercoaster. Because the brain's ability to regulate emotions and mood is influenced by estrogen levels, hormonal swings are a major factor in these variations in mood. It's critical to realize that these emotions are typical during the menopausal transition.

Techniques for Handling Emotional Swings

It helps to do things that encourage calmness and mental stability to deal with these emotional fluctuations. Exercise regularly, getting enough sleep, and practicing stress-reduction methods like yoga or meditation can help. Having a solid support system and, if necessary, obtaining professional assistance can also help to stabilize a person during emotionally turbulent times.

Increasing Fortitude and Discovering Joy

During menopause, cultivating resilience entails learning how to handle stress and adjust to changing circumstances. Living a resilient life can make you happier and possibly prolong your life. To build resilience, take care of yourself, find happy things to do, and keep an optimistic mindset.

Developing Contentment and Health

Focusing on the good things in life and partaking in fulfilling activities are key to finding joy during menopause. Engaging in a pastime, making connections with friends, or just spending some time for oneself can all help to improve mood and foster happiness and well-being.

This chapter sheds light on the emotional side of menopause and offers helpful tips for overcoming mood swings and developing resilience so that you can enjoy this life-changing time.

Chapter 7

Social Dynamics

Changes in Relationships and Communication Techniques

A phase of adjustment in interpersonal relationships may coincide with menopause. Effective communication is increasingly more important during this period since it facilitates navigating potential emotional and physical changes.

Recognizing the Changes

Changes in mood and energy levels during menopause can affect relationships with friends, family, and partners. Patience and understanding can be promoted by recognizing these changes and having an honest discussion about them.

Techniques for Powerful Communication

Using techniques like active listening, openly expressing wants and feelings, and setting boundaries can help preserve and improve relationships. These methods can aid in establishing an atmosphere that is encouraging to both sides.

Building a Community of Support

During menopause, a supportive group can be a lifesaver, offering a sense of understanding and connection.

Expanding Your Connections

Reaching out to friends, joining support groups, or taking part in community events can all help build a network of support. These relationships can provide a sense of shared camaraderie, emotional support, and helpful advice.

Having Conversations with Peers

It might be especially consoling to connect with those who are experiencing similar things. Sharing personal experiences, advice, and encouragement is made possible, and this can be quite helpful during this period of transition.

Chapter 8

Intimacy and Sexual Health

Recognizing and Adjusting to Libido Shifts

A frequent experience for many women is changes in libido brought on by menopause. A decrease in sex drive may be caused by a drop in hormone levels, especially those of estrogen and testosterone. This chapter explores the psychological and physiological elements that lead to these modifications and provides coping mechanisms.

Physical Factors Affecting Libido

Menopause-related hormonal changes can cause physical symptoms like a dry vagina and pain during intercourse, which can lower one's desire for sexual relations. Finding solutions, like utilizing lubricants or looking into more comfortable ways of sexual expression, starts with understanding these physical changes.

Psychological and Emotional Aspects

Sexual health and emotional well-being are intimately related. Menopause can occasionally cause depressive or insecure sentiments, which can lower libido. Taking care of these psychological issues is equally as crucial as treating physical ailments.

Increasing Closeness: Useful Advice and Methods

With the appropriate strategy, intimacy can be preserved and even improved during menopause. To assist women and their partners in navigating this new stage of their sexual relationship, this section offers helpful advice and strategies.

Interaction and Establishment

It's critical to be open and honest with your spouse about your needs and experiences. Talking about what works and what doesn't can foster a closer bond and understanding.

Discovering Novel Paths of Enjoyment

During menopause, creativity may be essential to sustaining a satisfying sexual life. Examining alternative forms of sex, such as massage or oral sex, can help you feel pleasure without any pain.

Lifestyle Factors to Take Into Account

Sexual desire can be increased by leading a healthy lifestyle that includes regular exercise and a balanced diet. This can also boost one's self-esteem. A positive self-image can lead to a more fulfilling sexual life.

Expert Assistance

Never be afraid to ask for help from medical professionals or therapists who specialize in sexual health. They can provide direction and individualized treatment plans.

Chapter 9

Postmenopausal Life

Long-Term Health Issues to Take Into Account

Following menopause, women must take care of several long-term health issues. It is essential to comprehend this to preserve health and avoid issues.

Heart Conditions

Because their estrogen levels are decreased after menopause, women are more likely to develop heart disease. It's critical to control cholesterol, and blood pressure, and lead a heart-healthy lifestyle.

Density of Bones

Osteoporosis risk is raised by the reduction in estrogen, which also affects bone density. It is advised to get regular bone density tests and to eat a diet high in calcium and vitamin D.

Menopause's Genitourinary Syndrome (GSM)

A variety of symptoms involving the urinary and genital systems, including dryness and incontinence, are included in GSM. Talking to a healthcare professional about symptoms is crucial because there are treatments available.

Getting Ready for a Bright Future

With the appropriate attitude to health and lifestyle, life after menopause can be bright and rewarding.

Exercise and Diet

A healthy postmenopausal lifestyle is built on a balanced diet and consistent activity. They support mood enhancement, weight management, and bone and muscle strength maintenance.

Frequent Medical Examinations

It's critical to keep up with medical screenings. Routine examinations can identify problems early on when they are most easily treated.

Mental Health

Both physical and health are equally important. A person's quality of life can be improved by participating in social events, pursuing hobbies, and asking for help when needed.

An outline of the most important health factors to think about after menopause is given in this chapter, along with tips for making plans for a healthy future. Women can have a healthy, active post-menopausal life by addressing these issues.

Chapter 10

Tales of Rejuvenation

Motivational Narratives of Development and Change

Menopause is the start of a new stage of life with many opportunities for development and change, not only the cessation of reproduction. This section features motivational tales of women who overcame menopause obstacles to become stronger and more contented.

Accepting Change

Women with a variety of backgrounds describe how they accepted the changes that menopause brought about. Numerous people gained a greater appreciation for life, while some uncovered untapped abilities and others found new careers.

Development Above Symptoms

Menopause can be a complicated journey, but it also offers chances for growth on the inside. These stories demonstrate how women have overcome their symptoms to discover happiness and a new purpose in their post-menopausal years.

Proven Advice for Living a Whole Life After Menopause

It's possible to experience bright health and vitality after menopause. Professionals offer advice on how to make the most of this phase of life.

Well-being and Health

Sustaining a wholesome way of living is essential for prospering after menopause. A healthy diet, consistent exercise, and mental health treatment are regarded by experts as the cornerstones of a high quality of life.

Sustained Development and Education

The years following menopause are a great period for personal development and education. To make the most of their postmenopausal years, experts advise women to take up new hobbies, continue their education throughout their lives, and be involved in society.

Optimistic outlook

A positive mindset can make a big difference in how someone experiences menopause and beyond. To promote a more fulfilling life after menopause, experts advise concentrating on the advantages, such as being free of the menstrual cycle and experiencing a newfound sense of liberation.

CONCLUSION

Every woman is affected differently by the menopause, which is a big life transformation. This trip, which is frequently accompanied by mental and physical changes, can be difficult, but it also offers chances for development and rejuvenation. We have discussed the many facets of menopause in this book, including the early warning signs and symptoms, coping mechanisms, and the significance of preserving both physical and mental health.

As we come to an end, it's critical to keep in mind that menopause is both a beginning and a finish. It's the perfect time to take control of your health, welcome change with confidence, and feel optimistic about the future. The years following menopause can be among the most active and satisfying of your life provided you have the correct information, encouragement, and mindset.

Accept this shift with an open mind and heart, and proceed knowing that you have the knowledge and skills necessary to handle this normal stage of life with courage and grace. Menopause is a trip, and like with all journeys, the experiences along the way are just as important as the final destination.